HIIT Your Way to a Slimmer, Stronger You

Harness the Power of High-Intensity Interval Training (HIIT) to Achieve Rapid Weight Loss, Build Muscle, and Enhance Overall Fitness

Brawn Babe

Table of Contents

Introduction

Welcome, fearless reader, to a journey that promises not just a slimmer, stronger you but a life-altering transformation fueled by the electrifying force of High-Intensity Interval Training, HIIT. Brace yourself, because we're about to embark on a fitness odyssey that goes beyond the mundane, shattering the confines of traditional workouts and unlocking the true potential within you.

Picture this: a workout so potent it leaves you breathless, muscles quivering, and endorphins soaring. That, my friend, is the magic of HIIT, a symphony of sweat, determination, and the sweet taste of victory. But this isn't just about getting fit; it's about tapping into the wellspring of strength you never knew existed.

In the pages that follow, we won't bore you with fitness jargon or one-size-fits-all solutions. Instead, we'll dive headfirst into the exhilarating world of HIIT, demystifying the science, sharing success stories, and arming you with the tools to sculpt your physique and elevate your well-being.

Imagine this book as your trainer, your confidant, and your kick-in-the-pants motivator, all rolled into one. We won't judge you for that secret love affair with pizza or the occasional Netflix binge, because let's face it, life is meant to be enjoyed. What we will do is empower you to conquer your fitness goals with gusto, injecting a dose of humor and wit into every burpee and squat.

This is not just about losing pounds; it's about gaining confidence, resilience, and a mindset that screams, "I can do anything." So, if you've ever felt the burn of frustration, the sting of self-doubt, or the longing for change, you're in the right place. Together, we'll turn those feelings into the fuel that propels you toward a slimmer, stronger, and more vibrant version of yourself.

Buckle up, champion. Your HIIT adventure begins now.

Your trainer, your confidant, and your kick-in-the-pants motivator, all rolled into one.

Chapter 1

Understanding High-Intensity Interval Training (HIIT)

The Science Behind HIIT

Picture yourself in a dimly lit laboratory, where scientists in white coats are unraveling the secrets of a fitness phenomenon that's changing lives, High-Intensity Interval Training, or as we affectionately call it, HIIT. But fear not, dear reader, you won't need a Ph.D. to grasp the science of this transformative exercise method. Let's break it down into bite-sized, sweat-worthy chunks.

The Anatomy of HIIT: A Symphony of Intensity and Rest

In the world of fitness, HIIT is the rockstar that knows how to hit the high notes. It's not just about mindlessly pounding the pavement or lifting heavy things; it's about strategic bursts of effort followed by sweet, sweet rest. Imagine a sprinter exploding off the blocks, then gracefully slowing down before the next burst. That, my friend, is the essence of HIIT.

EPOC: The Afterburn Effect

Now, let's talk about a little something called Excess Post-Exercise Oxygen Consumption (EPOC). It's not as intimidating as it sounds; in fact, it's your secret weapon for burning calories even after the workout is over. Think of it like this: after a HIIT session, your body is a metabolic furnace, torching calories to restore itself to its pre-exercise state. Translation? You're still melting away fat while catching your breath on the couch post-workout.

HIIT and Your Heart: A Love Story

Ah, the heart, the epicenter of your body's love affair with HIIT. As you push yourself to the limit, your heart races to keep up. This isn't just cardio; it's a symphony that strengthens your most vital muscle. With each interval, you're enhancing your cardiovascular fitness, reducing the risk of heart disease, and turning your ticker into a powerhouse.

Building Muscle, Torching Fat: The Dynamic Duo

HIIT isn't just about shedding pounds; it's sculpting lean muscle like Michelangelo with a chisel. Traditional cardio might bid adieu to muscle mass as it burns fat, but not HIIT. This dynamic duo preserves your hard-earned muscles while incinerating the unwanted fat layers, leaving you with a physique that's both powerful and defined.

Practical Tips for HIIT Success

Now that we've uncovered the HIIT masterpiece, let's talk practicality. To maximize your HIIT experience, consider these tips:

1. Start Slow: Rome wasn't built in a day, and neither is your HIIT prowess. Begin with manageable intervals and gradually ramp up the intensity.

2. Listen to Your Body: HIIT is about pushing limits, but not at the expense of your well-being. If your body signals a timeout, honor it.

3. Mix It Up: Variety is the spice of life, and the same goes for your workouts. Keep your routine exciting by introducing different exercises and intervals.

4. Fuel Smart: Your body is a high-performance machine, so treat it like one. Prioritize nutritious pre-and post-workout meals to optimize your results.

Congratulations! You've just graduated from HIIT Science 101. Armed with this knowledge, you're ready to dive into the heart-pounding, calorie-torching world of HIIT with confidence and zeal. In the next chapter, we'll explore the tangible benefits of HIIT for weight loss, muscle building, and overall fitness. Get ready to witness the magic unfold!

Benefits of HIIT for Weight Loss

Welcome to the chapter where we unveil the superhero cape that High-Intensity Interval Training (HIIT) wears when it comes to shedding those stubborn pounds. Imagine a workout that not only torches calories during the session but continues to incinerate fat long after you've caught your breath. This, my friend, is the magic of HIIT, and the benefits for weight loss are nothing short of extraordinary.

1. Igniting the Calorie Bonfire

In the realm of weight loss, it's all about calories in versus calories out. HIIT turns up the heat on this equation by creating a calorie bonfire. Those short, intense bursts of effort send your body into overdrive, demanding an immediate surge in energy. The result? You burn more calories in a shorter time than traditional workouts could ever dream of.

2. Afterburn Effect: Your 24/7 Fat Furnace

Prepare to be amazed by the Excess Post-Exercise Oxygen Consumption (EPOC), aka the Afterburn Effect. Long after your HIIT session concludes, your body is working tirelessly to restore itself. This means you're still shedding calories, turning your daily activities into mini fat-burning marathons. It's like having a personal fat furnace that operates 24/7.

3. Metabolic Makeover: Turning Fat into Fuel

HIIT isn't just about shedding pounds; it's a metabolic makeover. With each explosive interval, you're signaling to your body that it needs to become more efficient at using fat for fuel. Your metabolism kicks into high gear, becoming a lean, mean, fat-burning machine—even when you're enjoying that post-workout smoothie.

4. Preserving Lean Muscle Mass

Traditional weight loss methods often lead to a frustrating loss of muscle mass along with fat. Not HIIT. This superhero workout is designed to preserve your hard-earned muscles while targeting fat stores. You're not just losing weight; you're sculpting a lean, toned physique that's ready for the spotlight.

5. Hormonal Harmony: Taming the Fat-Storing Beast

HIIT plays a masterful tune with your hormones, especially the ones responsible for fat storage. It regulates insulin and leptin, making your body a less friendly environment for fat storage. It's like telling your hormones, "Hey, let's be friends with benefits, weight loss benefits!"

Practical Tips for Maximizing Weight Loss with HIIT

Now that you're ready to embrace the weight-loss wonders of HIIT, consider these practical tips:

1. Consistency is Key: Make HIIT a regular part of your routine for sustained results.

2. Challenge Yourself: As your fitness level improves, gradually increase the intensity to keep the fat-burning flames alive.

3. Combine HIIT with a Balanced Diet: Amplify your results by pairing HIIT with a nutrition plan that supports your weight loss goals.

4. Stay Hydrated: Water is the unsung hero of weight loss. Keep yourself hydrated to optimize your body's fat-burning capabilities.

5. Listen to Your Body: If an exercise feels too strenuous, modify it. The goal is progress, not injury.

With the benefits of HIIT for weight loss unveiled, it's time to lace up those workout shoes and dive into a fitness journey that not only transforms your physique but empowers you to embrace a healthier, more vibrant life. In the next chapter, we'll explore how HIIT builds muscle, turning you into a powerhouse of strength and endurance. Get ready to unleash your inner warrior!

Muscle Building with HIIT

Prepare to witness the marriage of intensity and muscle in a symphony of strength. High-Intensity Interval Training (HIIT) isn't just about shedding pounds; it's about sculpting lean, powerful muscles that tell a story of resilience and determination. In this chapter, we'll unravel the secrets behind HIIT's muscle-building prowess and guide you on a journey to transform your body into a fortress of strength.

1. The HIIT Blueprint for Muscle Growth

Contrary to the myth that lifting heavy weights is the sole path to muscle hypertrophy, HIIT introduces a refreshing twist. By incorporating explosive bursts of activity, HIIT triggers muscle fibers to adapt and grow. It's like sending an invitation to your muscles, saying, "Time to party, and you're the VIP guest!"

2. The Magic of Resistance: Against the Odds

HIIT isn't just about cardio; it's about resistance too. By integrating bodyweight exercises or adding resistance during intervals, you're challenging your muscles in ways that traditional workouts can't match. The result? A body that not only performs like a well-oiled machine but looks the part too.

3. Metabolic Overdrive: Burning Fat, Building Muscle

Here's the kicker: HIIT isn't just torching fat; it's building muscle simultaneously. Traditional cardio might be waving goodbye to your hard-earned muscles as it burns calories, but not HIIT. Your body becomes a multitasking marvel, sculpting lean muscle mass while incinerating fat layers. It's like getting a two-for-one deal on your fitness goals.

4. Fast-Twitch, Slow-Twitch: All Muscles Welcome

HIIT doesn't discriminate, it welcomes all muscles to the party. Whether you're activating fast-twitch muscles for explosive movements or engaging slow-twitch muscles for endurance, HIIT ensures a comprehensive workout that leaves no muscle fiber unturned. Say goodbye to imbalances and hello to a well-rounded physique.

5. Hormonal Harmony: The Muscle-Building Orchestra

Enter the orchestra of hormones, with HIIT as the conductor. Growth hormone and testosterone, the maestros of muscle building, take center stage during and after HIIT sessions. They're not just supporting your muscle growth; they're composing a symphony of strength that echoes long after your workout is complete.

Practical Tips for Maximizing Muscle Building with HIIT

Now that you're ready to sculpt a body that radiates strength, consider these practical tips:

1. Diversify Your Exercises: Target different muscle groups with a variety of exercises to ensure comprehensive development.

2. Progressive Overload: Gradually increase the intensity or resistance to keep challenging your muscles and promoting growth.

3. Recovery Matters: Give your muscles the love they deserve with proper rest and recovery to avoid burnout and maximize gains.

4. Fuel Smart: Provide your muscles with the nutrients they need by consuming a balanced diet rich in protein, carbohydrates, and healthy fats.

5. Celebrate Small Wins: Recognize and celebrate your muscle-building victories, whether it's lifting a heavier weight or mastering a challenging exercise.

With this newfound knowledge, you're equipped to embark on a journey that not only transforms your physique but instills a sense of empowerment and pride. The next chapter will delve into how HIIT enhances cardiovascular fitness, turning you into a cardiovascular powerhouse. Get ready to witness your heart leading the charge in the grand symphony of fitness!

Chapter 2

Getting Started with HIIT

Preparing for Your HIIT Journey

Welcome to the gateway of your High-Intensity Interval Training (HIIT) adventure, where the journey to a slimmer, stronger you begin. In this chapter, we'll delve into the essential preparations for your HIIT expedition, ensuring you step onto the path of transformation with confidence, enthusiasm, and a game plan designed for success.

1. Understanding Your WHY: The North Star of Your HIIT Journey

Before you break a sweat, take a moment to reflect on why you're embarking on this HIIT adventure. Is it to shed those persistent pounds, build muscle, or enhance overall fitness? Knowing your "why" will serve as your North Star, guiding you through the highs and lows of your fitness journey. Whether it's fitting into your favorite jeans or reclaiming your energy, a clear purpose fuels your motivation.

2. Assessing Your Fitness Level: A Reality Check

HIIT is for everyone, but not every HIIT workout fits every individual. Conduct an honest assessment of your current fitness level to tailor your HIIT experience accordingly. This evaluation isn't about judgment; it's about setting a baseline from which you can measure progress. Consider factors like stamina, strength, and any pre-existing health conditions to customize your HIIT approach.

3. Setting Realistic Goals: The Blueprint for Success

Dream big, but start small. Setting realistic, achievable goals is the blueprint for HIIT success. Break down your overarching fitness aspirations into manageable milestones. Whether it's completing a 20-minute session without gasping for air or mastering a new exercise, these mini-triumphs will fuel your motivation and propel you toward the grand finale.

4. Gathering the Right Gear: Your HIIT Arsenal

HIIT is the epitome of simplicity, but a few essentials can enhance your experience. Invest in comfortable, moisture-wicking workout attire, supportive footwear, and perhaps a timer or HIIT app to keep track of intervals. With the right gear in your arsenal, you'll be ready to conquer each HIIT session with focus and determination.

5. *Creating Your HIIT Space: Where Transformation Unfolds*

Transform any space into your personal HIIT sanctuary. Whether it's a corner of your living room or a patch of the great outdoors, designate an area where you can unleash your energy without distractions. Your HIIT space is not just physical; it's a mental space where you leave behind the stresses of the day and fully engage in the transformative power of HIIT.

Practical Tips for Preparing Your HIIT Journey

1. Start Slow: Rome wasn't built in a day, and neither is your HIIT prowess. Begin with manageable intervals and gradually ramp up the intensity.

2. Warm-Up Rituals: Prioritize a dynamic warm-up to prepare your body for the intensity ahead. This could include light cardio, dynamic stretches, and joint mobility exercises.

3. Know Your Limits: Listen to your body and respect its signals. If an exercise feels too challenging or if you experience pain, modify or take a break.

4. Hydrate: Water is your workout ally. Stay hydrated before, during, and after your HIIT session to optimize performance and recovery.

5. Celebrate Milestones: Acknowledge and celebrate even the smallest victories on your HIIT journey. Whether it's completing a challenging workout or improving your endurance, each step forward is a triumph.

With these preparations in place, you're not just starting a workout routine; you're embarking on a transformative journey. In the next chapter, we'll delve into the nitty-gritty of designing effective HIIT workouts tailored to your fitness goals. Get ready to unleash the power within!

Assessing Your Fitness Level

Before diving into the exhilarating world of High-Intensity Interval Training (HIIT), it's crucial to embark on your journey with a clear understanding of your current fitness landscape. Assessing your fitness level isn't about comparison or judgment; it's about creating a roadmap tailored to your unique strengths, challenges, and aspirations. Let's embark on this self-discovery expedition together.

1. *The Cardiovascular Check: Testing Your Endurance Horizon*

Begin by assessing your cardiovascular endurance, the engine that powers your body through the highs and lows of physical activity. Take note of how long you can sustain moderate-intensity activities like brisk walking, jogging, or cycling. If you find yourself easily winded or struggling to maintain a consistent pace, don't fret—this is your starting point.

2. *Strength Evaluation: Unearthing Your Power Potential*

Strength forms the bedrock of your fitness journey. Assess your current strength by gauging your ability to perform basic bodyweight exercises like squats, push-ups, or lunges. Take note of the number of repetitions and the level of effort required. Whether you can complete a set effortlessly or find it challenging, this insight will guide your initial approach to strength-focused HIIT exercises.

3. *Flexibility and Mobility: The Forgotten Dimensions*

Flexibility and mobility are the unsung heroes of overall fitness. Gauge your range of motion by attempting simple stretches or yoga poses. Are you able to touch your toes with ease, or does it feel like reaching for the stars? Assessing your flexibility provides valuable insights into potential areas of improvement and helps tailor your HIIT routine to enhance overall mobility.

4. *Listen to Your Body: The Ultimate Fitness Barometer*

Numbers and measurements are valuable, but the most critical assessment tool is your body itself. Take note of any discomfort, pain, or areas of weakness during physical activities. If a certain movement feels challenging or causes discomfort, it's a signal from your body. Listen attentively, respect these signals, and use them to customize your HIIT routine for a safe and effective fitness journey.

5. *Assessing Progress: The Ongoing Fitness Diary*

Fitness is a journey, not a destination. Regularly reassess your fitness level to track progress and adjust your HIIT routine accordingly. Celebrate victories—no matter how small, and use setbacks as learning opportunities. This ongoing assessment ensures that your fitness compass remains accurate, guiding you toward continuous improvement and success.

Practical Tips for Fitness Assessment

1. Record Baseline Measurements: Document initial performance levels in cardiovascular endurance, strength, and flexibility to establish a baseline for comparison.

2. Consult a Professional: If possible, seek guidance from a fitness professional or healthcare provider for a comprehensive assessment, especially if you have pre-existing health conditions.

3. Use a Fitness App or Journal: Keep a workout journal or use a fitness app to log your progress, making it easier to track improvements and adjust your HIIT routine.

4. Reassess Periodically: Aim for regular reassessments, perhaps every 4-6 weeks, to evaluate changes in your fitness levels and adjust your HIIT workouts accordingly.

5. Celebrate Improvements: Acknowledge and celebrate improvements, whether it's an increased number of push-ups, longer running intervals, or enhanced flexibility. Positive reinforcement fuels motivation.

As you navigate this fitness assessment journey, remember that everyone's starting point is unique. The key is not where you begin, but the direction in which you're heading. Armed with this self-awareness, you're ready to design a personalized HIIT experience that aligns with your fitness goals and sets the stage for a transformative adventure. In the next chapter, we'll delve into the art of setting realistic goals, paving the way for a purpose-driven HIIT journey. Get ready to define success on your terms!

Setting Realistic Goals

In the realm of High-Intensity Interval Training (HIIT), success isn't just about the destination; it's about the journey. Setting realistic goals provides the roadmap for this transformative expedition, ensuring that each step forward is purposeful, achievable, and deeply rewarding. Let's dive into the art of goal setting, crafting a narrative that propels you toward a slimmer, stronger version of yourself.

1. Dream Big, Start Small: The Power of Incremental Progress

Your fitness journey is an evolving masterpiece, and realistic goals form the brushstrokes that bring it to life. Dream big, envisioning the ultimate version of yourself, but break those aspirations into manageable, bite-sized goals. Whether it's completing a full HIIT session without rest or achieving a specific number of repetitions, these smaller victories lay the foundation for your grand triumph.

2. Specific, Measurable, Attainable, Relevant, Time-Bound (SMART): Your Goal Blueprint

Craft your goals with precision using the SMART framework. Make them Specific, clear and concise. Ensure they're Measurable, allowing you to track progress. Keep them Attainable, ambitious but realistic. Ensure they're Relevant to your overarching vision. Finally, set a Time frame, instilling a sense of urgency and accountability. The SMART framework transforms vague aspirations into tangible, actionable milestones.

3. Celebrate Progress, Embrace Setbacks: The Balanced Equation

Progress is a mosaic of achievements and setbacks. Celebrate each victory, whether it's completing an extra interval or mastering a new exercise. Equally important, embrace setbacks as learning opportunities, adjusting your goals and strategies accordingly. The journey is as much about resilience as it is about triumph.

4. Listen to Your Body: A Vital Goal Setting Principle

Your body is an eloquent communicator. Incorporate its signals into your goal-setting process. If you're consistently fatigued, adjust intensity or duration. If you're surpassing expectations, consider setting more challenging goals. Listening to your body ensures that your goals align with your current fitness level, fostering sustainable progress.

5. Long-Term Vision: Beyond the Finish Line

While setting short-term goals is vital, cultivating a long-term vision that transcends immediate achievements. Envision the lifestyle you aim to sustain, the habits you wish to embrace, and the enduring health benefits of your HIIT journey. This overarching vision serves as a guiding star, propelling you beyond the finish line toward a life of vitality and well-being.

Practical Tips for Goal Setting

1. Start with Clarity: Clearly define your overarching fitness objectives, then break them down into smaller, achievable goals.

2. Document Your Goals: Write down your goals in a journal or use a fitness app to track progress and stay accountable.

3. Regularly Evaluate: Periodically reassess your goals, adjusting them based on your evolving fitness level and aspirations.

4. Celebrate Achievements: Acknowledge and celebrate each milestone, reinforcing the positive behaviors that lead to success.

5. Stay Flexible: Life is dynamic, and so is your fitness journey. Be flexible in adapting your goals to accommodate unexpected challenges or opportunities.

With your goals set, you're not just embarking on a fitness journey; you're crafting a narrative of personal triumphs and transformative achievements. The next section explores safety precautions and common mistakes to ensure your HIIT adventure is not only exhilarating but also injury-free. Let's dive into the essentials of safe and effective training.

Safety Precautions and Common Mistakes

Before you lace up your workout shoes and dive headfirst into the pulsating world of High-Intensity Interval Training (HIIT), let's explore the essential safety precautions that will be your guiding lights. In this chapter, we'll navigate the potential pitfalls, ensuring your HIIT journey is not only invigorating but also injury-free.

1. Consultation with a Healthcare Professional: The Fitness Checkpoint

Before donning your workout gear, it's prudent to consult with a healthcare professional, especially if you have pre-existing health conditions. This crucial checkpoint ensures that your body is ready for the demands of HIIT, minimizing the risk of complications during intense workouts.

2. Warm-Up Rituals: The Gateway to Safe HIIT

The warm-up is your ticket to a safe and effective HIIT session. Engage in dynamic stretches, light cardio, and joint mobility exercises to prepare your body for the upcoming intensity. Skipping the warm-up not only increases the risk of injury but also hampers your performance during the workout.

3. Form Over Speed: The Golden Rule of HIIT

In the fervor of HIIT, it's easy to prioritize speed over form. However, maintaining proper form is paramount. Incorrect form not only diminishes the effectiveness of your workout but also elevates the risk of injury. Focus on executing each movement with precision, even if it means slowing down initially.

4. Gradual Progression: The Stepping Stones to Success

HIIT is a journey, not a sprint. Gradually progress the intensity and duration of your workouts to allow your body to adapt. Sudden, drastic changes increase the likelihood of overuse injuries and burnout. Listen to your body, and progress at a pace that aligns with your fitness level.

5. Hydration and Nutrition: Fueling Your Success

HIIT demands energy, and proper hydration and nutrition are the fuel that powers your success. Ensure you're adequately hydrated before, during, and after your workouts. Consume a balanced meal or snack that includes carbohydrates, protein, and fats to provide sustained energy for your session.

6. Recovery Rituals: The Post-HIIT Symphony

Recovery is an integral part of the HIIT equation. Allow your body time to rest and recuperate between sessions. Prioritize sleep, incorporate active recovery days, and listen to any signs of overtraining, such as persistent fatigue or muscle soreness.

Common Mistakes to Avoid: Navigating the HIIT Landscape

1. Ignoring Form for Speed: Sacrificing form for speed increases the risk of injury and compromises the effectiveness of your workout.

2. Overtraining: HIIT is intense, but more isn't always better. Overtraining can lead to burnout, fatigue, and increased susceptibility to injuries.

3. Skipping Warm-Up and Cool Down: Neglecting these crucial components increases the risk of injury and impairs recovery.

4. Inadequate Hydration: Dehydration hampers performance and increases the risk of heat-related issues. Hydrate consistently throughout your HIIT journey.

5. Lack of Adaptation: Failing to adapt your workouts to your fitness level can lead to overuse injuries. Customize your sessions based on your capabilities.

Practical Tips for Safe HIIT Training

1. Know Your Limits: Be mindful of your fitness level and progress gradually. Pushing beyond your limits increases injury risk.

2. Invest in Proper Footwear: Ensure your shoes provide adequate support, especially for high-impact activities in HIIT.

3. Listen to Your Body: If you experience persistent pain, discomfort, or unusual fatigue, it's a signal to reassess and modify your workouts.

4. Cross-Train: Incorporate a variety of exercises to prevent overuse injuries and ensure balanced muscle development.

5. Quality Over Quantity: Focus on the quality of your movements rather than the quantity. Each repetition should be deliberate and controlled.

By adhering to these safety precautions and avoiding common pitfalls, you're not just safeguarding your well-being; you're paving the way for a sustainable and rewarding HIIT journey. In the next chapters, we'll delve into the intricacies of crafting effective HIIT workouts and explore the multifaceted benefits that await you on this path of fitness discovery. Get ready to elevate your workout experience and achieve transformative results!

***Incorrect form not only
diminishes the effectiveness of
your workout but also elevates
the risk of injury.**￼*

Chapter 3

Designing Your HIIT Workouts

Customizing HIIT for Your Body

Now that you've set the stage with clear goals and safety precautions, it's time to step into the architect's shoes and design HIIT workouts tailored to your unique body and aspirations. This chapter unveils the art of crafting effective and personalized HIIT sessions that maximize results while honoring your strengths and challenges. Let's embark on this journey of customization, where each workout becomes a masterpiece sculpted for your success.

1. Know Your Body: The Blueprint for Customization

Understanding your body is the foundation of effective customization. Consider your fitness level, any pre-existing injuries, and areas of strength or weakness. If you're unsure, start with a basic HIIT routine and progressively customize it as you become more familiar with your body's response to different exercises.

2. Tailor Intervals to Your Fitness Level: The Goldilocks Principle

HIIT is about finding the sweet spot, the Goldilocks zone of intensity. Customize your intervals based on your fitness level. If you're a beginner, start with longer rest periods and shorter work intervals. As you progress, gradually decrease rest and increase intensity. Your goal is to push yourself without compromising form or safety.

3. Exercise Selection: The Art of Inclusion and Modification

Choose exercises that align with your fitness goals and accommodate any physical limitations. If an exercise feels challenging, consider modifications to reduce intensity while maintaining proper form. The beauty of HIIT lies in its versatility; feel free to swap exercises to keep your routine exciting and engaging.

4. Listen to Your Body During Workouts: Real-Time Customization

Your body is an eloquent communicator, even during the intensity of a HIIT session. If an exercise causes discomfort or if you're feeling fatigued, modify or skip it. Pay attention to signals of overexertion or potential injury, and adjust your intensity accordingly. HIIT is about pushing limits, but always with respect for your body's feedback.

5. Progressive Overload: Elevate Your HIIT Experience

As your body adapts to the demands of HIIT, introduce progressive overload to keep the challenge alive. This can include increasing the intensity, duration, or complexity of exercises. Gradual progression ensures continued improvements and prevents plateaus in your fitness journey.

6. Cross-Training for Comprehensive Fitness: HIIT's Dynamic Dance

Cross-training is the secret ingredient to a well-rounded HIIT routine. Integrate a variety of exercises to target different muscle groups and energy systems. This not only prevents boredom but also reduces the risk of overuse injuries. Balance high-impact exercises with low-impact alternatives to promote joint health.

Practical Tips for Customizing HIIT Workouts

1. Start with a Baseline: Begin with a basic HIIT routine and progressively customize based on your experience and comfort level.

2. Keep It Varied: Rotate exercises regularly to prevent monotony and ensure a balanced workout for all muscle groups.

3. Modify Intensity: Adjust the intensity of your HIIT sessions based on your energy levels, sleep quality, and overall well-being.

4. Incorporate Rest Days: Allow your body to recover by scheduling rest or active recovery days. Overtraining can hinder progress.

5. Document and Evaluate: Keep a workout journal or use a fitness app to document your HIIT sessions. Regularly evaluate what works and what needs adjustment.

By customizing your HIIT workouts to suit your body's needs and capabilities, you're not just exercising; you're engaging in a tailored fitness experience that aligns with your goals and promotes long-term success. In the upcoming chapters, we'll explore the diverse benefits of HIIT, from weight loss and muscle building to cardiovascular health. Get ready to witness the multifaceted impact of your personalized HIIT journey!

Choosing the Right Exercises

Selecting the right exercises is the artistry behind a successful High-Intensity Interval Training (HIIT) routine. Each exercise is a brushstroke, contributing to the masterpiece of your fitness journey. In this chapter, we'll explore the types of exercises that harmonize with the principles of HIIT, ensuring an engaging, effective, and well-rounded workout experience.

1. Cardiovascular Exercises: Igniting the Metabolic Flames

Cardiovascular exercises form the backbone of many HIIT sessions, elevating your heart rate and firing up your metabolism. Incorporate dynamic, full-body movements that engage large muscle groups. Examples include:

Sprinting: Whether on a track, treadmill or in an open space, short bursts of sprinting are classic HIIT cardio.

Jumping Jacks: An excellent way to raise your heart rate, engage your lower body, and add a touch of nostalgia to your routine.

Mountain Climbers: Combining core engagement with cardio, mountain climbers are a dynamic addition to any HIIT workout.

2. *Strength Training Exercises: Building a Foundation of Power*

Strength training in HIIT isn't about lifting heavy weights for extended periods; it's about explosive, controlled movements that engage multiple muscle groups. These exercises contribute to muscle building and overall strength. Examples include:

Bodyweight Squats: A fundamental lower body exercise, squats activate your quadriceps, hamstrings, and glutes.

Push-Ups: Engaging the chest, shoulders, and triceps, push-ups are a versatile upper body strength exercise.

Dumbbell Thrusters: Combining a squat with an overhead press, dumbbell thrusters offer a full-body strength and cardio challenge.

3. *Plyometric Exercises: Unleashing Explosive Power*

Plyometric exercises involve quick, powerful movements to build explosive strength. These exercises often incorporate jumping and are excellent for enhancing athletic performance. Examples include:

Box Jumps: Jumping onto a box or platform engages your lower body muscles and challenges your coordination.

Burpees: A full-body exercise that combines a squat, plank, and jump, burpees are a potent plyometric move.

Jump Lunges: Alternating jumping lunges target your legs while also working on balance and agility.

4. Core Exercises: The Powerhouse Foundation
A strong core is crucial for stability and overall functional fitness. Incorporate core exercises to enhance balance and support other movements. Examples include:

Plank Variations: Standard planks, side planks, and plank jacks engage your core muscles.

Russian Twists: Seated or standing, this exercise targets your obliques, enhancing rotational strength.

Leg Raises: Lying on your back, leg raises activate your lower abdominal muscles.

5. Active Recovery Exercises: Sustaining Momentum
Active recovery exercises help maintain a level of activity during rest intervals, keeping your heart rate elevated and promoting calorie burn. Examples include:

Marching in Place: Lift your knees alternately while standing in place to sustain a low-intensity workout.

Light Jogging or Walking: A gentle jog or brisk walk during rest intervals helps maintain circulation without exhaustive effort.

Dynamic Stretching: Incorporate dynamic stretches like leg swings or arm circles to enhance flexibility and prepare your body for the next high-intensity interval.

Practical Tips for Exercise Selection in HIIT
1. Consider Your Fitness Level: Choose exercises that align with your current fitness level and gradually progress as your strength and endurance improve.

2. Mix and Match: Variety keeps your workout exciting and engages different muscle groups. Combine cardio, strength, plyometric, and core exercises for a comprehensive session.

3. Adapt to Your Environment: Whether at home, the gym, or outdoors, select exercises that suit your available space and equipment.

4. Listen to Your Body: If an exercise causes pain or discomfort beyond normal fatigue, modify or replace it to prevent injury.

5. Customize for Goals: Tailor your exercise selection based on your fitness goals. If weight loss is a priority, emphasize cardiovascular exercises. If muscle building is the focus, incorporate more strength training moves.

By selecting a diverse range of exercises that align with your fitness goals and preferences, you're not just working out; you're crafting a personalized, dynamic HIIT experience that keeps you engaged and motivated. In the following chapters, we'll explore the benefits of these exercises in-depth, uncovering the transformative impact they can have on weight loss, muscle building, and overall fitness. Get ready to witness the magic of a well-chosen HIIT routine!

Structuring an Effective HIIT Session

Designing a High-Intensity Interval Training (HIIT) session is akin to orchestrating a symphony—each element harmonizing to create a powerful, transformative experience. In this chapter, we'll break down the key components of structuring an effective HIIT session, ensuring that every interval, every movement, contributes to the crescendo of your fitness journey.

1. Warm-Up: Tuning Your Body for Action
The warm-up is the overture, setting the stage for the intensity that follows. Engage in dynamic stretches, light cardio, and joint mobility exercises to gradually elevate your heart rate and prepare your muscles for the upcoming challenge. A well-tuned warm-up not only reduces the risk of injury but also enhances the effectiveness of the ensuing workout.

2. Interval Structure: The Heartbeat of HIIT
HIIT is characterized by alternating intervals of high-intensity exercise and periods of rest or lower-intensity activity. The interval structure is the heartbeat of your session, and its design depends on your fitness goals. Common structures include:

Tabata: 20 seconds of intense exercise followed by 10 seconds of rest, repeated for four minutes.

1:1 Ratio: Equal time for high-intensity exercise and rest, such as 30 seconds on, and 30 seconds off.

Pyramid: Gradually increasing and then decreasing the duration or intensity of intervals.

3. Exercise Selection: The Instruments of Intensity

Choose a diverse range of exercises that align with your goals and target different muscle groups. Mix cardiovascular, strength, plyometric, and core exercises to create a comprehensive workout. Ensure each exercise is performed with proper form and intensity. Rotate exercises regularly to prevent boredom and target various muscle groups.

4. Intensity Levels: Finding Your Fortissimo

Intensity is the soul of HIIT. Each high-intensity interval should push you to your limits, whether through speed, resistance, or effort. The goal is to work at an intensity that challenges your cardiovascular and muscular systems. Listen to your body, aim for an 8-9 on a perceived exertion scale of 1-10, and progressively increase intensity as your fitness improves.

5. Rest and Recovery: Breathing Between Movements

Rest intervals are not breaks; they're the pauses between movements, allowing your body to recover and prepare for the next burst of intensity. The length of rest depends on your fitness level and the structure of your session. Use this time to regulate your breathing, hydrate, and mentally prepare for the next round.

6. Cool Down: The Serenade to Soothe

As your HIIT symphony concludes, transition into a cooldown to ease your body back to a resting state. Incorporate static stretches that target the muscles used during the session. This helps prevent muscle stiffness, improves flexibility, and promotes recovery.

7. Hydration and Nutrition: The Fuel for Your Fitness Opera

Proper hydration and nutrition play vital roles in the success of your HIIT session. Hydrate adequately before, during, and after your workout. Consume a balanced meal or snack that includes carbohydrates, protein, and healthy fats to fuel your energy demands.

Practical Tips for Effective HIIT Sessions

1. Plan and Prepare: Outline your session in advance, including exercise selection, interval structure, and desired intensity levels.

2. Progress Gradually: If you're new to HIIT, start with shorter sessions and lower intensity. Gradually increase as your fitness improves.

3. Listen to Your Body: Pay attention to how your body responds during and after each session. Adjust your plan based on your individual needs and feedback.

4. Include Variety: Keep your sessions engaging by introducing new exercises, interval structures, or workout formats.

5. Record and Reflect: Keep a workout journal to document your sessions, noting what worked well and areas for improvement.

By meticulously structuring your HIIT sessions, you're not just exercising; you're crafting a symphony of intensity that propels you toward your fitness goals. In the upcoming chapters, we'll explore the specific benefits of HIIT for weight loss, muscle building, and overall health, providing a deeper understanding of the transformative power embedded in each interval. Get ready to witness the impact of your well-structured HIIT routine!

Incorporating Variety for Long-Term Success

Variety is the spice that keeps your High-Intensity Interval Training (HIIT) journey vibrant, engaging, and sustainable. In this chapter, we'll explore the importance of incorporating variety into your HIIT routine and how it contributes to long-term success, ensuring that each workout remains exciting, effective, and adaptive to your evolving fitness needs.

1. Battling Boredom: The Enemy of Consistency

Repeating the same HIIT routine day in and day out can lead to boredom, diminishing your enthusiasm and motivation. Variety introduces a sense of novelty, transforming each session into a new and exciting challenge. This freshness not only keeps you mentally engaged but also encourages consistency by making your workouts something to look forward to.

2. Targeting Different Muscle Groups: Balanced Development

Each exercise in your HIIT repertoire places a unique demand on specific muscle groups. Incorporating variety ensures that you target different muscles, promoting balanced development throughout your body. This comprehensive approach helps prevent overuse injuries, enhances overall strength, and contributes to a well-rounded physique.

3. Avoiding Plateaus: The Pitfall of Predictability

The human body is remarkably adaptive. Performing the same exercises repeatedly can lead to plateaus, where your progress stagnates as your body becomes accustomed to the routine. By introducing variety, you challenge your muscles in new ways, preventing plateaus and promoting continuous improvement. This dynamic approach is key to unlocking your body's full potential.

4. Adapting to Fitness Levels: Inclusivity for All

HIIT is for everyone, regardless of fitness level. Incorporating a variety of exercises allows for inclusivity, ensuring that individuals with different fitness levels and abilities can participate. Beginners can start with lower-impact movements, gradually progressing to more intense exercises. Meanwhile, those with advanced fitness can continue to challenge themselves with complex and demanding movements.

5. Mental Stimulation: A Workout for Your Brain

HIIT isn't just a physical challenge; it's a mental one as well. The cognitive engagement required to learn and perform new exercises stimulates your brain, enhancing the overall mental benefits of your workout. The continuous learning curve keeps your mind sharp and your interest piqued, fostering a positive mindset toward your fitness journey.

6. Fun Factor: Enjoyment Fuels Consistency

Variety injects an element of fun into your HIIT sessions. Whether it's trying a new exercise, exploring different workout formats, or incorporating group activities, the enjoyment factor plays a crucial role in sustaining long-term consistency. When your workouts are enjoyable, you're more likely to stick with them, creating a positive feedback loop for continued success.

Practical Tips for Incorporating Variety into Your HIIT Routine

1. Rotate Exercises Regularly: Change your exercise selection every few weeks to keep things interesting and target different muscle groups.

2. Explore Different Formats: Experiment with various HIIT formats, such as circuit training, interval running, or AMRAP (As Many Rounds As Possible) workouts.

3. Include Outdoor Workouts: Take your HIIT sessions outdoors to enjoy a change of scenery and the benefits of natural elements.

4. Try New Equipment: Incorporate different equipment like resistance bands, kettlebells, or medicine balls to add variety and intensity to your workouts.

5. Participate in Classes or Group Sessions: Joining classes or group sessions introduces you to new exercises and fosters a sense of community.

Chapter 4

Nutrition for HIIT Success

Fueling Your Workouts

Nutrition is the silent ally that fuels the fire of your High-Intensity Interval Training (HIIT) sessions. In this chapter, we'll explore the critical role of nutrition in optimizing your HIIT performance, ensuring that you have the energy, endurance, and recovery support necessary to push your limits and achieve success in each exhilarating session.

1. Pre-Workout Nutrition: Energizing the Engine

Before embarking on a HIIT adventure, it's essential to provide your body with the right fuel. Pre-workout nutrition aims to enhance energy levels and prepare your muscles for the demands of high-intensity exercise. Consider the following guidelines:

Timing: Consume a balanced meal or snack containing carbohydrates, protein, and a small amount of healthy fats 1-2 hours before your HIIT session.

Carbohydrates: Choose complex carbohydrates such as whole grains, fruits, and vegetables. These provide a steady release of energy during your workout.

Protein: Include a moderate amount of protein to support muscle function and repair. Options like yogurt, lean meats, or plant-based protein sources are ideal.

Hydration: Begin your workout well-hydrated. Drink water throughout the day and consider sipping on a small amount of water leading up to your session.

2. During Your HIIT Session: Staying Hydrated

HIIT sessions can be intense, leading to increased sweat and potential dehydration. Staying properly hydrated during your workout is crucial for maintaining performance and preventing fatigue. Consider the following hydration tips:

Water Intake: Sip water consistently during your HIIT session, especially during rest intervals. Small, frequent sips are more effective than large gulps.

Electrolytes: For longer or particularly intense sessions, consider a sports drink or coconut water to replenish electrolytes lost through sweat.

3. Post-Workout Nutrition: Recovery and Repair

The post-workout window is a critical period for replenishing glycogen stores, repairing muscle tissue, and kickstarting recovery. Tailor your post-workout nutrition to support these processes:

Timing: Consume a post-workout meal or snack within 30 minutes to an hour after your HIIT session to optimize recovery.

Carbohydrates: Include carbohydrates to replenish glycogen stores. Opt for a mix of simple and complex carbohydrates for a quick energy boost and sustained replenishment.

Protein: Prioritize protein intake to support muscle repair and growth. Sources like lean meats, dairy, eggs, or plant-based proteins are excellent choices.

Hydration: Continue to hydrate post-workout to replace fluids lost during the session.

4. Individualized Nutrition: Listening to Your Body

Nutritional needs vary among individuals based on factors such as age, gender, metabolism, and overall health. Pay attention to how your body responds to different foods and adjust your nutrition plan accordingly. Experiment with timing, macronutrient ratios, and food choices to discover what works best for you.

5. *Supplements for HIIT: Enhancing Performance*

While a well-balanced diet should be the primary source of nutrients, supplements can complement your nutrition plan, especially if you have specific goals or dietary restrictions. Consider consulting with a healthcare professional or nutritionist before incorporating supplements. Common supplements for HIIT enthusiasts may include:

Protein Powder: A convenient way to boost protein intake, particularly if it's challenging to meet your protein goals through whole foods.

BCAAs (Branched-Chain Amino Acids): These amino acids support muscle recovery and may be beneficial for those engaging in frequent and intense exercise.

Electrolyte Supplements: Useful for individuals who engage in prolonged or intense workouts, especially in hot environments.

Practical Tips for Optimal Nutrition in HIIT

1. Listen to Hunger Signals: Pay attention to your body's hunger and fullness cues. Eat when hungry and stop when satisfied.

2. Balance Macronutrients: Ensure your meals include a balance of carbohydrates, proteins, and healthy fats for sustained energy and recovery.

3. Whole Foods First: Prioritize whole, nutrient-dense foods over processed options. These provide a broader range of essential nutrients.

4. Experiment and Adjust: Nutrition is highly individual. Experiment with different approaches and adjust based on how your body responds.

5. Stay Consistent: Consistency is key in nutrition. Aim for a balanced and varied diet consistently to support your overall health and fitness goals.

By aligning your nutrition with the demands of your HIIT sessions, you're not just fueling your workouts; you're laying the groundwork for enhanced performance, faster recovery, and long-term success. In the next chapters, we'll delve into the specific benefits of HIIT for weight loss, muscle building, and cardiovascular health, providing a comprehensive understanding of the transformative power embedded in each interval. Get ready to witness the profound impact of a well-nourished and energized HIIT journey!

Pre- and Post-Workout Nutrition

In the dynamic world of High-Intensity Interval Training (HIIT), strategic nutrition is your secret weapon. This chapter delves into the intricacies of pre-and post-workout nutrition, guiding you on how to optimize your energy levels, enhance performance, and promote effective recovery for a successful HIIT journey.

1. Pre-Workout Nutrition: Priming the Engine

Fueling your body before a HIIT session is akin to priming the engine before a race. The right combination of nutrients ensures that you have the energy and stamina to tackle the intensity of your workout. Consider the following pre-workout nutrition strategies:

Timing is Key: Consume a balanced meal or snack 1-2 hours before your HIIT session to allow for proper digestion. If you're short on time, opt for a smaller snack 30 minutes before.

Carbohydrates for Energy: Include complex carbohydrates like whole grains, fruits, or vegetables. These provide a steady release of energy during your workout.

Moderate Protein Intake: Incorporate a moderate amount of protein to support muscle function and repair. Greek yogurt, lean meats, or plant-based protein sources are excellent choices.

Hydration Matters: Begin your workout well-hydrated. Drink water throughout the day, and consider sipping on a small amount of water leading up to your session.

2. During Your HIIT Session: Staying Hydrated and Energized

HIIT sessions can be intense, and maintaining hydration and energy levels during the workout is crucial for sustained performance. Consider the following tips:

Hydration is Continuous: Sip water consistently during your HIIT session, especially during rest intervals. Small, frequent sips are more effective than large gulps.

Consider Electrolytes: For longer or particularly intense sessions, consider a sports drink or coconut water to replenish electrolytes lost through sweat.

3. Post-Workout Nutrition: The Key to Recovery and Growth

The post-workout period is a critical window for recovery, replenishing glycogen stores, and kickstarting muscle repair. Tailor your post-workout nutrition to maximize these processes:

Timing is Crucial: Consume a post-workout meal or snack within 30 minutes to an hour after your HIIT session to optimize recovery.

Carbohydrates for Glycogen Replenishment:
Include carbohydrates to replenish glycogen stores.
Simple carbohydrates provide a quick energy boost,
while complex carbohydrates sustain replenishment.

Prioritise Protein Intake: Protein is essential for
muscle repair and growth. Prioritize protein sources
such as lean meats, dairy, eggs, or plant-based options.

Hydrate for Recovery: Continue to hydrate
post-workout to replace fluids lost during the session.

4. Individualized Approach: Listening to Your Body

Nutritional needs vary among individuals based on
factors such as age, gender, metabolism, and overall
health. Pay attention to how your body responds to
different foods and adjust your nutrition plan
accordingly. Experiment with timing, macronutrient
ratios, and food choices to discover what works best for
you.

5. Supplements for Support: Enhancing Performance

While whole foods should be the primary source of
nutrients, supplements can complement your nutrition
plan, especially for specific goals or dietary restrictions.
Consider the following:

Protein Powder: A convenient way to boost protein intake, especially if meeting protein goals through whole foods is challenging.

BCAAs (Branched-Chain Amino Acids): These amino acids support muscle recovery and may be beneficial for those engaging in frequent and intense exercise.

Electrolyte Supplements: Useful for individuals participating in prolonged or intense workouts, particularly in hot environments.

Practical Tips for Optimal Pre- and Post-Workout Nutrition

1. Plan Ahead: Schedule your meals and snacks to ensure proper pre-and post-workout nutrition, especially if you have a busy schedule.

2. Balance Macronutrients: Include a mix of carbohydrates, proteins, and healthy fats in both your pre-and post-workout meals for comprehensive nutritional support.

3. Whole Foods First: Prioritize whole, nutrient-dense foods over processed options for a broad spectrum of essential nutrients.

4. Experiment and Adjust: Nutrition is highly individual. Experiment with different approaches and adjust based on how your body responds.

5. Stay Consistent: Consistency is key in nutrition. Aim for a balanced and varied diet consistently to support your overall health and fitness goals.

By fine-tuning your pre-and post-workout nutrition, you're not just fueling your HIIT sessions; you're unlocking the potential for heightened performance, faster recovery, and long-term success. In the following chapters, we'll explore the specific benefits of HIIT for weight loss, muscle building, and cardiovascular health, providing a comprehensive understanding of the transformative power embedded in each interval. Get ready to witness the profound impact of a well-nourished and energized HIIT journey!

-

Hydration Tips for HIIT

Hydration is the unsung hero of High-Intensity Interval Training (HIIT), playing a pivotal role in sustaining energy levels, preventing fatigue, and supporting overall performance. In this chapter, we'll dive into essential hydration tips to ensure you're adequately fueled and ready to conquer the intensity of your HIIT sessions.

1. Start Hydrated: Lay the Foundation

Begin your HIIT journey well-hydrated. Proper hydration starts long before you hit the workout mat or start your sprint intervals. Consistently drink water throughout the day to maintain baseline hydration levels. This initial foundation sets the stage for a more effective and energized HIIT experience.

2. Pre-Workout Hydration: Sip Strategically

Optimal hydration before your HIIT session is crucial for performance. Consider these pre-workout hydration tips:

Timing is Key: Drink water 1-2 hours before your workout to allow for adequate fluid absorption without causing discomfort during exercise.

Monitor Urine Color: Aim for pale yellow urine, indicating that you are well-hydrated. Darker urine may suggest dehydration.

Avoid Overhydration: While staying hydrated is essential, avoid excessive water intake just before your workout, as this can lead to discomfort and potentially disrupt your session.

3. Hydrate During HIIT: Sip Smartly

During your HIIT session, maintaining fluid balance is vital to prevent dehydration and sustain performance. Consider these hydration strategies:

Small, Frequent Sips: Instead of consuming large amounts of water at once, sip water consistently during your workout, especially during rest intervals.

Electrolyte Considerations: For longer or more intense sessions, consider drinks containing electrolytes to replace those lost through sweat. Sports drinks or coconut water are suitable options.

Listen to Your Thirst: Trust your body's signals. If you feel thirsty, take a sip. Thirst is an early sign of dehydration.

4. Post-Workout Hydration: Recovery Refuel

After the HIIT storm, prioritize replenishing lost fluids to support recovery. Follow these post-workout hydration tips:

Prompt Rehydration: Consume water or a hydrating beverage within 30 minutes to an hour after your workout to kickstart the recovery process.

Electrolyte Replenishment: If you've engaged in a particularly intense or prolonged session, consider replenishing electrolytes with a sports drink or natural sources like fruits.

5. Individual Hydration Needs: Personalize Your Approach

Hydration is not one-size-fits-all. Factors such as body weight, sweat rate, climate, and individual differences influence hydration needs. Pay attention to how your body responds to different hydration strategies and customize your approach accordingly.

6. Hydration Beyond Water: Diversify Your Intake

While water is the primary hydrator, incorporate hydrating foods into your diet. Fruits and vegetables with high water content, such as watermelon, cucumber, and oranges, contribute to your overall fluid intake.

Practical Tips for Effective Hydration in HIIT

1. Establish a Routine: Create a hydration routine that aligns with your daily schedule and workout times.

2. Carry a Water Bottle: Keep a water bottle with you throughout the day and during your workout for easy access to hydration.

3. Educate Yourself: Learn about your individual hydration needs by monitoring urine color, paying attention to thirst cues, and experimenting with different hydration strategies.

4. Monitor Sweat Rate: Weigh yourself before and after a workout to estimate your sweat rate. For every pound lost, aim to drink about 16-24 ounces of fluid.

5. Consider Weather Conditions: Adjust your hydration plan based on the climate. Hot and humid conditions may require increased fluid intake.

By prioritizing proper hydration, you're not just preventing dehydration; you're optimizing your body's ability to perform at its peak during HIIT. In the upcoming chapters, we'll explore the specific benefits of HIIT for weight loss, muscle building, and cardiovascular health, providing a comprehensive understanding of the transformative power embedded in each interval. Get ready to witness the profound impact of a well-hydrated and energized HIIT journey!

Chapter 5

Tracking Progress and Staying Motivated

Setting Up a HIIT Journal

Embarking on a High-Intensity Interval Training (HIIT) journey is not just about physical exertion; it's a holistic experience that encompasses progress tracking and unwavering motivation. In this chapter, we'll explore the importance of monitoring your progress and staying motivated, introducing the invaluable tool of a HIIT journal to guide you on this transformative path.

1. The Power of Progress Tracking

Progress tracking is the compass that keeps you on course during your HIIT expedition. Whether your goal is weight loss, muscle building, or overall fitness enhancement, monitoring your progress provides tangible evidence of your journey's success. Consider the following aspects for effective progress tracking:

Fitness Metrics: Record key metrics such as weight, body measurements, and body fat percentage at regular intervals. These metrics offer insights into your body's physical transformations.

Workout Performance: Track the intensity, duration, and types of exercises in each HIIT session. Note any increases in weights, improved completion times, or enhanced endurance.

Energy Levels and Recovery: Document how you feel before, during, and after workouts. Assess your energy levels, mood, and recovery rate. This information helps fine-tune your approach for optimal performance.

2. The Motivational Impact of Progress

Witnessing tangible progress serves as a powerful motivator, propelling you forward in your HIIT journey. As you flip through your journal and observe improvements, both big and small, you'll find renewed motivation to conquer each session and strive for your overarching fitness goals.

3. The Role of a HIIT Journal

A HIIT journal serves as your chronicle, capturing the nuances of your fitness expedition. Here's how to set up and maximize the benefits of your HIIT journal:

Choose Your Format: Select a format that suits your preferences, whether it's a physical notebook, a digital document, or a specialized fitness app. The key is to make it a tool that seamlessly integrates into your routine.

Establish Baseline Measurements: Begin your journal by documenting baseline measurements, including weight, body measurements, and fitness assessments. These initial entries set the stage for future comparisons.

Record Workout Details: After each HIIT session, log the specifics of your workout. Include details such as exercise types, duration, intensity levels, and any modifications or challenges faced. This information provides a blueprint for future workouts.

Capture Personal Reflections: Dedicate a section for personal reflections. Note how you felt during the workout, any mental or emotional insights, and your overall satisfaction with the session. This reflective space enhances mindfulness and self-awareness.

Set Short-Term and Long-Term Goals: Outline specific, measurable, and time-bound goals in your journal. Break them down into short-term and long-term objectives. Regularly revisit and update these goals as you progress.

Celebrate Achievements: Take a moment to celebrate milestones and achievements. Whether it's completing a challenging workout, reaching a weight-loss goal, or improving your overall fitness, acknowledging your accomplishments fuels positive reinforcement.

4. Staying Motivated Beyond the Journal

While a HIIT journal is a potent motivational tool, staying inspired goes beyond written entries. Consider additional strategies to keep the flames of motivation burning:

Variety in Workouts: Inject variety into your HIIT routine to prevent monotony. Experiment with different exercises, formats, and environments to keep things exciting.

Connect with the HIIT Community: Engage with the broader HIIT community through social media, fitness forums, or local fitness groups. Share your journey, gain inspiration from others, and foster a sense of camaraderie.

Reward System: Establish a reward system for achieving specific milestones. Treat yourself to a small indulgence or plan a special activity as a reward for your hard work and dedication.

Regular Assessments: Conduct regular assessments of your progress, adjusting your goals and workout strategies as needed. The ongoing evaluation ensures that your HIIT journey remains aligned with your evolving fitness aspirations.

Practical Tips for Successful Progress Tracking and Motivation

1. Consistency is Key: Regularly update your HIIT journal. Consistent entries provide a comprehensive overview of your journey.

2. Be Honest and Transparent: Record both successes and challenges in your journal. Honest documentation creates a realistic portrayal of your progress.

3. Visual Aids: Include visual aids such as progress photos or charts to enhance the visual representation of your journey.

4. Review and Reflect: Set aside time to review your journal and reflect on your achievements. This reflective practice reinforces your commitment and dedication.

5. Share Your Journey: Consider sharing your HIIT journey with a workout buddy, coach, or friends. Accountability and support from others can amplify your motivation.

By integrating progress tracking and motivation strategies into your HIIT routine, you're not just exercising; you're engaging in a transformative journey that extends beyond physical fitness.

Measuring Performance Improvements

In the realm of High-Intensity Interval Training (HIIT), the pursuit of progress is not just a desire, it's a cornerstone. This chapter is dedicated to unraveling the metrics that define your journey, offering insights into how to measure and celebrate the remarkable improvements that unfold as you conquer each interval.

1. The Essence of Performance Metrics

Performance metrics are the yardsticks by which you gauge your advancement in the world of HIIT. These metrics extend beyond the numbers on a scale; they encapsulate the multidimensional facets of your physical capabilities, endurance, and overall fitness. Here are key metrics to consider:

Weight and Body Composition:
Weight: Regularly weigh yourself to monitor changes over time. However, remember that weight alone does not reflect overall fitness.

Body Fat Percentage: A more accurate indicator of body composition. Tools like calipers or bioelectrical impedance scales can help track changes in fat percentage.

Endurance and Cardiovascular Fitness:
Duration: Record the time you can sustain high-intensity efforts. As your endurance improves, you'll notice longer periods of sustained effort.

Resting Heart Rate: A lower resting heart rate is often indicative of improved cardiovascular fitness. Measure your resting heart rate consistently, preferably upon waking.

Strength and Power:
Lifted Weight: For exercises involving weights, track the amount of weight lifted. Gradual increases indicate improved strength.

Repetition Counts: Note the number of repetitions completed for each exercise. Increasing repetitions or maintaining high counts signals improved muscular endurance.

Speed and Agility:
Sprint Times: If your HIIT includes sprinting, measure the time it takes to complete sprints. Improved speed signifies enhanced agility and cardiovascular capacity.

Reaction Time: For exercises involving rapid movements, track your reaction time. A decrease in reaction time indicates improved agility.

2. *The Importance of Consistent Tracking*

Consistency in tracking these metrics is paramount. Regular measurements provide a comprehensive view of your journey, allowing you to identify trends, patterns, and areas for improvement. Set a schedule for assessments, whether it's weekly, bi-weekly, or monthly, and adhere to it diligently.

3. *Celebrating Non-Numerical Achievements*

While numerical metrics are crucial, don't overlook the non-numerical victories that contribute to your overall success:

Improved Form: Notice enhancements in your exercise form. This indicates increased strength, stability, and muscle control.

Increased Range of Motion: If your exercises involve flexibility, observe improvements in your range of motion. Enhanced flexibility contributes to overall joint health and performance.

Mental Endurance: Take note of your mental resilience during workouts. As you progress, you'll likely find it easier to push through challenges and stay focused.

Adaptability: If you're incorporating new and challenging exercises, the ability to adapt and perform them more efficiently is a noteworthy accomplishment.

4. Adjusting Goals and Expectations

As you measure performance improvements, it's essential to adjust your goals and expectations accordingly:

Reassess and Set New Goals: Periodically reassess your goals based on your achievements. Set new, challenging objectives to maintain momentum.

Acknowledge Plateaus: Recognize that progress may not always be linear. Plateaus are natural, and they present opportunities to reassess your approach and make necessary adjustments.

5. The Holistic Picture of Progress

Remember that progress in HIIT is not solely defined by numbers. The holistic picture of progress encompasses physical, mental, and emotional dimensions. Feelings of increased energy, heightened mood, and a sense of accomplishment are all vital aspects of your journey.

6. Celebrating Milestones

Celebrate your milestones, whether big or small. Recognizing and celebrating achievements fosters a positive mindset, reinforcing your commitment to the HIIT journey.

Practical Tips for Measuring Performance Improvements

1. Create a Tracking System: Use a journal, spreadsheet, or fitness app to systematically record your metrics.

2. Consistency is Key: Perform assessments under similar conditions each time to ensure accurate and comparable results.

3. Seek Professional Guidance: Consider consulting with a fitness professional or healthcare provider for assistance in setting realistic goals and interpreting metrics.

4. Embrace the Non-Numerical Wins: Acknowledge and celebrate improvements in form, mental endurance, and adaptability.

5. Adjust Goals Appropriately: Regularly reassess your goals based on achievements and adapt them to your evolving capabilities.

By meticulously measuring and celebrating your performance improvements, you're not just tracking numbers; you're unveiling the profound transformations taking place within each interval.

Overcoming Plateaus

Plateaus are a natural part of any fitness journey, and High-Intensity Interval Training (HIIT) is no exception. This chapter is dedicated to helping you navigate and overcome plateaus, ensuring that stagnation becomes a mere stepping stone to renewed progress and achievement.

1. Understanding Plateaus

A plateau in your HIIT progress is a phase where you may experience a temporary halt or slowdown in performance improvement. This can manifest as a lack of changes in weight, diminished increases in strength, or a sense of stagnation in your workouts.

2. The Causes of Plateaus

Understanding the potential causes of plateaus is crucial for devising effective strategies to overcome them:

Adaptation: The body is exceptionally adaptive. Over time, it becomes accustomed to the stress placed on it during HIIT, leading to a plateau.

Overtraining: Excessive exercise without adequate recovery can lead to a plateau. Your body needs time to repair and adapt to the stress of high-intensity workouts.

Nutritional Factors: Inadequate nutrition can hinder progress. Ensure you're consuming the right balance of nutrients to support your HIIT efforts.

Lack of Variety: Performing the same exercises repeatedly can lead to plateaus. Your body may benefit from new challenges and varied movements.

3. Strategies for Overcoming Plateaus

Overcoming plateaus requires a multi-faceted approach, addressing both physical and mental aspects of your HIIT journey:

Change Your Routine:

Vary Your Exercises: Introduce new exercises or modify existing ones. This change challenges your body in different ways, preventing it from adapting too quickly.

Alter Intensity: Adjust the intensity of your HIIT sessions. You can increase the duration of high-intensity intervals, reduce rest periods, or incorporate more challenging movements.

Focus on Recovery:

Prioritize Rest: Ensure adequate rest between intense sessions. Overtraining can hinder progress, and sufficient rest allows your body to repair and strengthen.

Incorporate Active Recovery: Include active recovery days with low-intensity activities like walking, yoga, or swimming to maintain movement without excessive stress.

Nutritional Adjustments:

Reassess Your Diet: Evaluate your nutritional intake. Ensure you're consuming enough calories, macronutrients, and micronutrients to support your energy needs and recovery.

Consider Supplements: Consult with a healthcare professional or nutritionist to determine if supplements could address specific deficiencies or enhance your performance.

Set New Goals:
Reevaluate and Adjust Goals: Periodically reassess your short-term and long-term goals. Adjusting your objectives provides fresh targets to strive for, rekindling motivation.

Celebrate Non-Numerical Wins: Acknowledge and celebrate improvements in form, mental endurance, and overall well-being.

Monitor Stress Levels:
Assess External Stressors: External stressors, both physical and emotional, can impact your ability to progress. Evaluate and manage stress in other areas of your life.

Incorporate Stress-Reduction Techniques: Practice stress-reduction techniques such as meditation, deep breathing, or mindfulness to enhance overall well-being.

4. The Mental Aspect of Overcoming Plateaus

The psychological dimension is equally vital in overcoming plateaus:

Maintain a Positive Mindset: Plateaus are part of the journey. Embrace them as opportunities for growth rather than setbacks.

Stay Patient and Persistent: Progress takes time. Trust the process, stay persistent, and recognize that breakthroughs often come after periods of challenge.

Celebrate Small Wins: Acknowledge and celebrate small victories. Each step forward, no matter how modest, contributes to your overall success.

5. Practical Tips for Overcoming Plateaus
1. Regularly Assess Your Routine: Evaluate your workout routine to ensure it remains challenging and diverse.

2. Prioritize Recovery: Allow sufficient time for rest and recovery to prevent burnout.

3. Nutritional Evaluation: Assess your diet for adequacy and consider consulting a nutritionist for personalized guidance.
4. Set New Goals: Establish new, realistic goals to reignite motivation and focus.

5. Mind-Body Connection: Pay attention to how your body responds to workouts, and be mindful of stress levels.

6. Seek Support: Connect with a workout buddy, coach, or community for encouragement and advice.

Overcoming plateaus is an integral part of the dynamic journey that is HIIT. By implementing these strategies and maintaining a resilient mindset, you're not just breaking through boundaries; you're forging a path to sustained progress and success. In the following chapters, we'll explore the specific benefits of HIIT for weight loss, muscle building, and cardiovascular health, providing a comprehensive understanding of the transformative power embedded in each interval. Get ready to transcend plateaus and reach new heights in your HIIT journey!

Staying Inspired for the Long Haul

Embarking on a High-Intensity Interval Training (HIIT) journey is a commitment to your well-being, and the path to lasting success requires more than momentary motivation, it demands sustained inspiration. In this chapter, we'll explore strategies to kindle and maintain the flame of inspiration throughout the long and invigorating road of your HIIT expedition.

1. Cultivating Intrinsic Motivation
Intrinsic motivation, the inner drive that comes from within, forms the bedrock of enduring inspiration. To cultivate and sustain this intrinsic motivation:

Define Your "Why": Clarify your reasons for engaging in HIIT. Whether it's improving health, boosting energy, or achieving a specific fitness goal, a clear "why" serves as a constant source of inspiration.

Connect with Personal Values: Align your HIIT journey with your core values. When your actions resonate with your values, motivation becomes a natural byproduct.

Celebrate the Process: Shift the focus from outcome-based goals to the process of self-improvement. Embrace the small victories, relish the journey, and acknowledge progress as an ongoing pursuit.

2. Setting Realistic and Evolving Goals

Goals act as guideposts on your HIIT journey, providing direction and purpose. Ensure your goals are:

S.M.A.R.T.: Specific, Measurable, Achievable, Relevant, and Time-bound. Clearly defined goals create a roadmap, making your progress tangible and achievable.

Evolving: Regularly reassess and adjust your goals to reflect your evolving capabilities and aspirations. Setting new challenges prevents monotony and fosters ongoing motivation.

3. Building a Support System

Surrounding yourself with a supportive network enhances your resilience and motivation:

Workout Buddies: Join forces with a workout buddy or a community. Shared experiences and mutual encouragement create a sense of camaraderie, making the journey more enjoyable.

Professional Guidance: Consider consulting with a fitness coach or trainer. Expert guidance can provide personalized strategies, address challenges, and inject fresh perspectives into your routine.

Social Media Engagement: Connect with the broader fitness community through social media. Share your journey, gain inspiration from others, and contribute to a supportive online environment.

4. Embracing Variety and Novelty
Variety is the spice of life, and it's also a key ingredient in maintaining inspiration:

Diversify Your Workouts: Introduce new exercises, formats, or classes to keep your routine exciting. Novelty reignites enthusiasm and challenges your body in different ways.

Explore Outdoor Activities: Take your workouts outside. Whether it's hiking, cycling, or outdoor HIIT sessions, the change of scenery adds a refreshing dimension to your fitness routine.

5. Incorporating Mindfulness Practices
Mindfulness practices contribute to a centered and present mindset, enhancing overall well-being and sustaining inspiration:

Mindful Breathing: Incorporate mindful breathing exercises into your routine. Focusing on your breath can center your mind and enhance your connection with your body during workouts.

Yoga and Stretching: Integrate yoga or stretching sessions to promote flexibility, balance, and mindfulness. These practices complement the intensity of HIIT while fostering a holistic approach to fitness.

6. Celebrating Milestones and Acknowledging Efforts

Acknowledge and celebrate every milestone, regardless of size, and recognize the effort invested in your HIIT journey:

Keep a Success Journal: Record your achievements, big or small, in a success journal. Reflecting on your progress reinforces the positive aspects of your journey.

Reward System: Establish a reward system for reaching milestones. Treat yourself to a small indulgence or plan a special activity as a tangible acknowledgment of your efforts.

7. Periodic Reflection and Reframing

Periodically reflect on your journey, reframe challenges, and adjust your mindset:

Reflect on Progress: Regularly assess your progress and acknowledge the positive changes in your fitness, energy levels, and overall well-being.

Reframe Challenges: View challenges as opportunities for growth rather than setbacks. Embracing difficulties with a growth mindset fosters resilience and inspiration.

8. Finding Joy in Movement

Rediscover the joy in movement by connecting with activities that bring genuine happiness:

Explore Fun Workouts: Experiment with workouts that bring joy, whether it's dance, martial arts, or sports. Enjoying the process makes it easier to stay inspired.

Listen to Your Body: Pay attention to how your body responds to different forms of exercise. Choose activities that align with your preferences and bring a sense of fulfillment.

9. Patience and Long-Term Vision

Cultivate patience and embrace a long-term vision for your HIIT journey:

Practice Patience: Understand that progress takes time, and results may not always be immediately apparent. Consistent effort, combined with patience, yields lasting success.

Visualize Long-Term Health: Envision the long-term benefits of HIIT for your health and well-being. Focusing on the broader impact enhances motivation beyond immediate goals.

Practical Tips for Long-Term Inspiration

1. Morning Routine: Incorporate HIIT into your morning routine to set a positive tone for the day.

2. Mix Up Your Playlist: Create dynamic playlists to keep your workouts engaging and energizing.

3. Periodic Breaks: Schedule occasional breaks to prevent burnout and maintain enthusiasm.

4. Mindful Reflection: Dedicate time for mindful reflection on your fitness journey, acknowledging both challenges and achievements.

5. Plan Active Social Activities: Integrate social activities that involve movement, such as group hikes, outdoor sports, or fitness classes with friends.

By nurturing enduring inspiration, you're not just engaging in HIIT; you're fostering a lifelong commitment to your well-being. In the upcoming

The path to lasting success requires more than momentary motivation.

Chapter 6

HIIT for Specific Goals

Rapid Weight Loss Strategies

Embarking on a High-Intensity Interval Training (HIIT) journey opens the door to a myriad of fitness goals, and for many, rapid weight loss is a primary objective. This chapter will delve into tailored strategies within the HIIT framework that specifically target and accelerate the process of shedding unwanted pounds.

1. Understanding HIIT's Impact on Weight Loss

Before delving into strategies, it's essential to grasp why HIIT is a potent tool for rapid weight loss:

Elevated Caloric Burn: The intense bursts of activity during HIIT elevate the heart rate, leading to a higher caloric expenditure both during and after the workout, a phenomenon known as the afterburn effect or excess post-exercise oxygen consumption (EPOC).

Preservation of Lean Muscle Mass: Unlike traditional steady-state cardio, HIIT places a significant demand on the muscles. This demand encourages the preservation of lean muscle mass, crucial for a healthy metabolism.

Metabolic Boost: HIIT has been shown to enhance metabolic rate, contributing to increased calorie burning even at rest. This metabolic boost is instrumental in achieving and maintaining weight loss.

2. Structuring HIIT Workouts for Weight Loss

To optimize HIIT for rapid weight loss, consider the following structuring principles:

Interval Duration and Intensity: Short, intense intervals interspersed with brief rest periods are the hallmarks of effective HIIT for weight loss. Aim for intervals lasting 20-30 seconds at near-maximum effort, followed by 10-15 seconds of rest.

Variety in Exercises: Incorporate a diverse range of exercises to engage multiple muscle groups. This not only keeps workouts interesting but also ensures a comprehensive calorie burn.

Progressive Overload: Gradually increase the intensity of your HIIT workouts to continually challenge your body. This can involve increasing the intensity of exercises, duration of intervals, or incorporating more advanced movements.

3. Targeted Strategies for Rapid Weight Loss

High-Intensity Intervals:

Tabata Protocol: Adopt the Tabata method, consisting of 20 seconds of all-out effort followed by 10 seconds of rest, repeated for four minutes. This format maximizes calorie burn in a short time.

Pyramid Intervals: Gradually increase and then decrease the intensity and duration of intervals within a single workout. For example, start with 15 seconds, progress to 30 seconds, then decrease back down.

Combination Workouts:
Cardio-Resistance Fusion: Combine cardiovascular exercises with resistance training in a single HIIT session. This dual approach enhances calorie burn and promotes muscle development.

Circuit Training: Design HIIT circuits that incorporate both aerobic and strength exercises. This not only stimulates weight loss but also enhances overall fitness.

Interval Running:
Sprint Intervals: Incorporate sprint intervals into your running routine. Sprint at maximum effort for 20-30 seconds, followed by a slow jog or walk for recovery.

Hill Sprints: If possible, incorporate hill sprints into your outdoor workouts. The incline adds an extra challenge, intensifying calorie burn.

Bodyweight HIIT:
Bodyweight Exercises: Leverage the effectiveness of bodyweight exercises such as burpees, squat jumps, and mountain climbers. These compound movements engage multiple muscle groups, accelerating calorie expenditure.

HIIT Yoga: Integrate dynamic yoga poses into your HIIT routine. The combination of strength-building and flexibility enhances the overall weight loss impact.

4. Nutrition Strategies to Support Weight Loss HIIT

While exercise is a crucial component, nutrition plays an equally vital role in rapid weight loss. Consider these strategies:

Pre-Workout Nutrition: Consume a balanced meal or snack 1-2 hours before your HIIT session. Include a combination of carbohydrates and protein for sustained energy.

Post-Workout Nutrition: Optimize recovery by consuming a protein-rich meal or shake within 30 minutes of completing your HIIT workout. This aids in muscle repair and supports metabolism.

Hydration: Stay well-hydrated, as proper hydration supports overall metabolism and can contribute to a feeling of fullness, preventing overeating.

Caloric Deficit: To achieve rapid weight loss, create a caloric deficit by ensuring that your total caloric intake is lower than the calories burned through HIIT and other daily activities.

5. Consistency and Sustainability

Rapid weight loss is most effective when integrated into a sustainable and consistent routine:

Establish a Routine: Design a realistic and consistent workout schedule that aligns with your lifestyle. This fosters habit formation and long-term adherence.

Mindful Eating: Practice mindful eating by paying attention to hunger and fullness cues. This approach encourages a healthier relationship with food, supporting sustainable weight loss.

Rest and Recovery: Prioritize rest days to allow your body to recover. Overtraining can impede progress and hinder weight loss efforts.

Adapt to Preferences: Choose HIIT exercises that you enjoy. Enjoyment increases the likelihood of sustained commitment to your weight loss journey.

6. Monitoring Progress and Adjusting Strategies

Regular Assessments: Periodically reassess your weight loss goals and adjust your HIIT strategies accordingly. Adaptations may be needed as your body responds to the initial stages of weight loss.

Celebrate Milestones: Acknowledge and celebrate milestones along the way. Recognizing progress reinforces positive behaviors and fosters motivation.

By strategically incorporating HIIT into your weight loss journey, you're not just shedding pounds; you're sculpting a sustainable and healthy approach to fitness. In the following chapters, we'll explore the specific benefits of HIIT for muscle building, cardiovascular health, and overall well-being, providing a comprehensive understanding of the transformative power embedded in each interval. Get ready to witness the profound impact of targeted HIIT strategies on your rapid weight loss goals!

Conclusion

As we draw the curtains on this exploration of High-Intensity Interval Training (HIIT) and its transformative power, envision the journey ahead, where the pursuit of a slimmer, stronger you becomes a reality. Through the pages of this guide, we've navigated the science behind HIIT, delved into tailored strategies for weight loss, and uncovered the keys to unlocking your full fitness potential.

The road to fitness is not just a destination but an ongoing adventure, and HIIT serves as your steadfast companion on this voyage. As you harness the intensity of each interval, remember that every drop of sweat is a testament to your commitment, every challenge is an opportunity for growth, and every triumph is a step closer to the vibrant, healthier version of yourself.

So, armed with the knowledge within these pages, go forth and HIIT your way to a slimmer, stronger you. Let each interval be a declaration of your resilience, each workout a celebration of your dedication, and each achievement a testament to the extraordinary capabilities within you. Embrace the power of HIIT, and watch as it shapes not just your physique but the essence of who you are, a dynamic, empowered individual on the path to lasting well-being.

May the intensity of your commitment echo in the echoes of your achievements, and may the journey to a slimmer, stronger you be as invigorating as the intervals that propel you forward. This is not just a conclusion; it's an invitation to embrace the ongoing adventure of HIIT, a journey that promises not just physical transformation but a holistic renewal of mind, body, and spirit.

HIIT your way to a slimmer, stronger you, the journey continues, and the best is yet to come.